Plan

CookBook

90 Quick, Easy, and Delicious Vegetarian Recipes.
Weight Loss to start a Healthy Eating.

Eva Green

CONTENTS

CHAPTER 1: BREAKFASTS

1. Tasty Oatmeal Muffins

Preparation time: 10 minutes

Cooking time: 20 minutes

Servings: 12

Ingredients:

½ cup of hot water

½ cup of raisins

¼ cup of ground flaxseed

2 cups of rolled oats

¼ teaspoon of sea salt

½ cup of walnuts

¼ teaspoon of baking soda

1 banana

2 tablespoons of cinnamon

¼ cup of maple syrup

Directions:

Whisk the flaxseed with water and allow the mixture to sit for about 5 minutes.

In a food processor, blend all the ingredients along with the flaxseed mix. Blend everything for 30 seconds, but do not create a smooth substance. To create rough-textured cookies, you need to have a semi-coarse batter.

Put the batter in cupcake liners and place them in a muffin tin. As this is an oil-free recipe, you will need cupcake liners. Bake everything for about 20 minutes at 350 degrees.

Enjoy the freshly-made cookies with a glass of warm milk.

Nutrition: Calories: 133, Fats 2 g, Carbohydrates 27 g, Protein 3 g

2. Omelet with Chickpea Flour

Preparation time: 10 minutes

Cooking time: 20 minutes

Serving: 1

Ingredients:

½ teaspoon, onion powder

¼ teaspoon, black pepper

1 cup, chickpea flour

½ teaspoon, garlic powder

½ teaspoon, baking soda

¼ teaspoon, white pepper

1/3 cup, nutritional yeast

3 finely chopped green onions

4 ounces, sautéed mushrooms

Directions:

In a small bowl, mix the onion powder, white pepper, chickpea flour, garlic powder, black and white pepper, baking soda, and nutritional yeast.

Add 1 cup of water and create a smooth batter.

On medium heat, put a frying pan and add the batter just like the way you would cook pancakes.

On the batter, sprinkle some green onion and mushrooms. Flip the omelet and cook evenly on both sides.

Once both sides are cooked, serve the omelet with spinach, tomatoes, hot sauce, and salsa.

Nutrition: Calories: 150, Fats 1.9 g, Carbohydrates 24.4 g, Proteins 10.2 g

3. White Sandwich Bread

Preparation time: 10 minutes

Cooking time: 20 minutes

Servings: 16

Ingredients:

1 cup warm water

2 tablespoons active dry yeast

4 tablespoons oil

2 ½ teaspoons salt

2 tablespoons raw sugar or 4 tablespoons maple syrup /agave

nectar

1 cup warm almond milk or any other nondairy milk of your choice

6 cups all-purpose flour

Directions:

Add warm water, yeast and sugar into a bowl and stir. Set aside for 5

minutes or until lots of tiny bubbles are formed, sort of frothy.

Add flour and salt into a mixing bowl and stir. Pour the oil, yeast mix

and milk and mix into dough. If the dough is too hard, add a little

water, a tablespoon at a time and mix well each time. If the dough is

too sticky, add more flour, a tablespoon at a time. Knead the dough

for 8 minutes until soft and supple. You can use your hands or use the dough hook attachment of the stand mixer.

Now spray some water on top of the dough. Keep the bowl covered with a towel. Let it rest until it doubles in size.

Remove the dough from the bowl and place on your countertop. Punch the dough.

Line a loaf pan with parchment paper. You can also grease with ome oil if you prefer. You can use 2 smaller loaf pans if you want to make smaller loaves, like I did.

Place the dough in the loaf pan. Now spray some more water on top of the dough. Keep the loaf pan covered with a towel. Let it rest until the dough doubles in size.

Bake in a preheated oven at 370° F for about 40 – 50 minutes or a toothpick when inserted in the center of the bread comes out without any particles stuck on it.

Let it cool to room temperature.

Cut into 16 equal slices and use as required. Store in a breadbox at room temperature.

Nutrition: Calories 209, Fat 4 g, Carbohydrate 35 g, Protein 1 g

4. A Toast to Remember

Preparation time: 10 minutes

Cooking time: 15 minutes

Servings: 4

Ingredients:

1 can, black beans

Pinch, sea salt

2 pieces, whole-wheat toast

¼ teaspoon, chipotle spice

Pinch, black pepper

1 teaspoon, garlic powder

1 freshly juiced lime

1 freshly diced avocado

¼ cup, corn

3 tablespoons, finely diced onion

½ freshly diced tomato

Fresh cilantro

Directions:

Mix the chipotle spice with the beans, salt, garlic powder, and pepper. Stir in the lime juice.

Boil all of these until you have a thick and starchy mix.

In a bowl, mix the corn, tomato, avocado, red onion, cilantro, and juice from the rest of the lime. Add some pepper and salt.

Toast the bread and first spread the black bean mixture followed by the avocado mix.

Take a bite of wholesome goodness!

Nutrition: Calories: 290, Fats 9 g, Carbohydrates 44 g, Proteins 12 g

5. Tasty Panini

Preparation time: 5 minutes

Cooking time: 0 minutes

Serving: 1

Ingredients:

¼ cup, hot water

1 tablespoon, cinnamon

¼ cup, raisins

2 teaspoons, cacao powder

1 ripe banana

2 slices, whole-grain bread

¼ cup, natural peanut butter

Directions:

In a bowl, mix the cinnamon, hot water, raisins, and cacao powder.

Spread the peanut butter on the bread.

Cut the bananas and put them on the toast.

Mix the raisin mixture in a blender and spread it on the sandwich.

Nutrition: Calories: 850, Fats 34 g, Carbohydrates 112 g, Proteins 27 g

6. Tasty Oatmeal and Carrot Cake

Preparation time: 10 minutes

Cooking time: 10 minutes

Serving: 1

Ingredients:

1 cup, water

½ teaspoon, cinnamon

1 cup, rolled oats

Salt

¼ cup, raisins

½ cup, shredded carrots

1 cup, non-dairy milk

¼ teaspoon, allspice

½ teaspoon, vanilla extract

Toppings:

¼ cup, chopped walnuts

2 tablespoons, maple syrup

2 tablespoons, shredded coconut

Directions:

Put a small pot on low heat and bring the non-dairy milk, oats, and water to a simmer.

Now, add the carrots, vanilla extract, raisins, salt, cinnamon and allspice. You need to simmer all of the ingredients, but do not forget to stir them. You will know that they are ready when the liquid is fully absorbed into all of the ingredients (in about 7-10 minutes).

Transfer the thickened dish to bowls. You can drizzle some maple syrup on top or top them with coconut or walnuts.

Nutrition: Calories: 210, Fats 11.48 g, Carbohydrates 10.37 g, Proteins 3.8 g

7. Onion & Mushroom Tart with a Nice Brown Rice Crust

Preparation time 10 minutes

Cooking time 55 minutes

Serving: 1

Ingredients:

1 ½ pounds, mushrooms, button, portabella,

1 cup, short-grain brown rice

2 ¼ cups, water

½ teaspoon, ground black pepper

2 teaspoons, herbal spice blend

1 sweet large onion

7 ounces, extra-firm tofu

1 cup, plain non-dairy milk

2 teaspoons, onion powder

2 teaspoons, low-sodium soy

1 teaspoon, molasses

¼ teaspoon, ground turmeric

¼ cup, white wine

¼ cup, tapioca

Directions:

Cook the brown rice and put it aside for later use.

Slice the onions into thin strips and sauté them in water until they are soft. Then, add the molasses, and cook them for a few minutes.

Next, sauté the mushrooms in water with the herbal spice blend. Once the mushrooms are cooked and they are soft, add the white wine or sherry. Cook everything for a few more minutes.

In a blender, combine milk, tofu, arrowroot, turmeric, and onion powder till you have a smooth mixture

On a pie plate, create a layer of rice, spreading evenly to form a crust. The rice should be warm and not cold. It will be easy to work with warm rice. You can also use a pastry roller to get an even crust. With your fingers, gently press the sides.

Take half of the tofu mixture and the mushrooms and spoon them over the tart dish. Smooth the level with your spoon.

Now, top the layer with onions followed by the tofu mixture. You can smooth the surface again with your spoon.

Sprinkle some black pepper on top.

Bake the pie at 350o F for about 45 minutes. Toward the end, you can cover it loosely with tin foil. This will help the crust to remain moist.

Allow the pie crust to cool down, so that you can slice it. If you are in love with vegetarian dishes, there is no way that you will not love this

pie.

Nutrition: Calories: 245.3, Fats 16.4 g, Proteins 6.8 g, Carbohydrates

18.3 g

8. Perfect Breakfast Shake

Preparation time: 5 minutes

Cooking time: 0 minutes

Servings: 2

Ingredients:

3 tablespoons, raw cacao powder

1 cup, almond milk

2 frozen bananas

3 tablespoons, natural peanut butter

Directions:

Use a powerful blender to combine all the ingredients.

Process everything until you have a smooth shake.

Enjoy a hearty shake to kickstart your day.

Nutrition: Calories: 330, Fats 15 g, Carbohydrates 41 g, Proteins 11 g

9. Beet Gazpacho

Preparation time: 10 minutes

Cooking time: 2 minutes

Servings: 4

Ingredients:

½ large bunch young beets with stems, roots and leaves

2 small cloves garlic, peeled,

Salt to taste

Pepper to taste

½ teaspoon liquid stevia

1 glass coconut milk kefir

1 teaspoon chopped dill

½ tablespoon canola oil

1 small red onion, chopped

1 tablespoon apple cider vinegar

2 cups vegetable broth or water

1 tablespoon chopped chives

1 scallion, sliced

Roasted baby potatoes

Directions:

Cut the roots and stems of the beets into small pieces. Thinly slice the beet greens.

Place a saucepan over medium heat. Add oil. When the oil is heated, add onion and garlic and cook until onion turns translucent.

Stir in the beets, roots and stem and cook for a minute.

Add broth, salt and water and cover with a lid. Simmer until tender.

Add stevia and vinegar and mix well. Taste and adjust the stevia and vinegar if required.

Turn off the heat. Blend with an immersion blender until smooth.

Place the saucepan back over it. When it begins to boil, add beet greens and cook for a minute. Turn off the heat.

Cool completely. Chill if desired.

Add rest of the ingredients and stir.

Serve in bowls with roasted potatoes if desired.

Nutrition: Calories 101, Fats 5 g, Carbohydrates 14 g, Proteins 2 g

10. Vegetable Rice

Preparation time: 7 minutes

Cooking time: 15 minutes

Servings: 4

Ingredients:

½ cup brown rice, rinsed

1 cup water

½ teaspoon dried basil

1 small onion, chopped

2 tablespoons raisins

5 ounces frozen peas, thawed

½ cup pecan halves, toasted

1 medium carrot, cut into matchsticks

4 green onions, cut into 1-inch pieces

1 tablespoon olive oil

½ teaspoon salt or to taste

½ teaspoon crushed red chili flakes or to taste

Ground pepper or to taste

Directions:

Place a small saucepan with water over medium heat.

When it begins to boil, add rice and basil. Stir.

When it again begins to boil, lower the heat and cover with a lid.

Cook for 15 minutes until all the water is absorbed and rice is cooked. Add more water if you think the rice is not cooked well.

Meanwhile, place a skillet over medium high heat. Add carrots, raisins and onions and sauté until the vegetables are crisp as well as tender.

Stir in the peas, salt, pepper and chili flakes.

Add pecans and rice and stir.

Serve.

Nutrition: Calories 305, Fats 13 g, Carbohydrates 41 g, Proteins 8 g

11. Courgette Risotto

Preparation time: 10 minutes

Cooking time: 5 minutes

Servings: 8

Ingredients:

2 tablespoons olive oil

4 cloves garlic, finely chopped

1.5 pounds Arborio rice

6 tomatoes, chopped

2 teaspoons chopped rosemary

6 courgettes, finely diced

1 ¼ cups peas, fresh or frozen

12 cups hot vegetable stock

1 cup chopped

Salt to taste

Freshly ground pepper

Directions:

Place a large heavy bottomed pan over medium heat. Add oil. When the oil is heated, add onion and sauté until translucent.

Stir in the tomatoes and cook until soft.

Next stir in the rice and rosemary. Mix well.

Add half the stock and cook until dry. Stir frequently.

Add remaining stock and cook for 3-4 minutes.

Add courgette and peas and cook until rice is tender. Add salt and pepper to taste.

Stir in the basil. Let it sit for 5 minutes.

Nutrition: Calories 406, Fats 5 g, Carbohydrates 82 g, Proteins 14 g

12. Country Breakfast Cereal

Preparation Time: 5 minutes

Cooking time: 40 minutes

Servings: 6

Ingredients:

1 cup brown rice, uncooked

½ cup raisins, seedless

1 tsp cinnamon, ground

¼ Tbsp peanut butter

2 ¼ cups water

Honey, to taste

Nuts, toasted

Directions:

Combine rice, butter, raisins, and cinnamon in a saucepan. Add 2 ¼ cups water. Bring to boil.

Simmer covered for 40 minutes until rice is tender.

Fluff with fork. Add honey and nuts to taste.

Nutrition: Calories 160 Carbohydrates 34 g Fats 1.5 g Protein 3 g

13. Oatmeal Fruit Shake

Preparation Time: 10 minutes

Cooking time: 0 minutes

Servings: 2

Ingredients:

1 cup oatmeal, already prepared, cooled

1 apple, cored, roughly chopped

1 banana, halved

1 cup baby spinach

2 cups coconut water

2 cups ice, cubed

½ tsp ground cinnamon

1 tsp pure vanilla extract

Directions:

Add all ingredients to a blender.

Blend from low to high for several minutes until smooth.

Nutrition: Calories 270 Carbohydrates 58 g Fats 1.5 g Protein 5 g

14. Amaranth Banana Breakfast Porridge

Preparation Time: 10 minutes

Cooking time: 25 minutes

Servings: 8

Ingredients:

2 cup amaranth

2 cinnamon sticks

4 bananas, diced

2 Tbsp chopped pecans

4 cups water

Directions:

Combine the amaranth, water, and cinnamon sticks, and banana in a pot. Cover and let simmer around 25 minutes.

Remove from heat and discard the cinnamon. Places into bowls, and top with pecans.

Nutrition: Calories 330 Carbohydrates 62 g Fats 6 g Protein 10 g

15. Green Ginger Smoothie

Preparation time: 5 minutes

Cooking time: 5 minutes

Servings: 2

Ingredients:

1 banana

½ apple sliced

1 orange sliced and peeled

1 lemon juice

2 big spinach

1 tbsp. fresh ginger

½ cup almond milk

For the dressing: chia seeds, apple, raspberries

Directions:

Take a blender. Peel off and slice all fruits. Add banana, apple, orange, lime juice, ginger and spinach and blend them well until they turn smooth. Now add almond milk and pulse again for a few seconds. Pour the smoothie into glasses and serve. You can add chia seeds, apple or raspberries for a smoothie bowl. Store it up to 8-10 hours in the refrigerator.

Nutrition: Calories 330 Carbohydrates 62 g Fats 6 g Protein 10 g

16. Orange Dream Creamsicle

Preparation time: 5 minutes

Cooking time: 5 minutes

Servings: 2

Ingredients:

1 orange, peeled

¼ cup vegan yogurt

2 tbsp. orange juice

¼ tsp vanilla extract

4 ice cubes

Directions:

In a blender, add orange, orange juice, vegan yogurt, vanilla extract and ice cubes. Blend all the ingredients well until smooth and well combined. Pour it into smoothie glasses and serve.

Nutrition: Calories 120 Carbohydrates 62 g Fats 6 g Protein 10g

17. Strawberry Limeade

Preparation time: 5 minutes

Cooking time: 5 minutes

Servings: 6

Ingredients:

2 cup strawberries

1 cup sugar or as per taste

7 cups of water

2 cup lemon juice

Sliced berries for garnish

Directions:

Take a small bowl, add sugar and water and put in microwave until dissolved. Now take a blender and add strawberries and a cup of water and blend well. Combine the strawberries puree with the sugar dissolve water and mix. Pour lime juice and water if required. Stir well and chill before serving. You can add berries on the top as garnishing.

Nutrition: Calories; 144, carbohydrates: 37g, sugar: 35g

18. Peanut Butter and Jelly Smoothie

Preparation time: 5 minutes

Cooking time: 5 minutes

Servings: 2

Ingredients:

1 cup frozen raspberries

1 cup frozen strawberries

1 serving collagen peptides

1 tbsp. peanut butter

¾ cup almond milk

Directions:

Take a blender. Add in raspberries, strawberries, peanut butter, collagen peptide and almond milk. Blend all ingredients until well combined. Add almond milk as per the required consistency. Pour into smoothie serving glasses and top up with the peanut butter or anything of your choice for dressing.

Nutrition: Calories: 251, fat: 11.1g, carbohydrates: 27.5g, proteins: 15.7g

19. Banana Almond Granola

Preparation time: 10 minutes

Cooking time: 20 Minutes

Servings: 21

Ingredients:

Organic rolled whole oats – 3 Cups

Raw Almond – ½ Cup, chopped

Sunflower seeds – ½ Cup, raw

Vanilla Extract – ½ teaspoon

Sea salt – 1/8 teaspoon

Coconut oil – 3 tablespoons, organic

Honey – 3 tablespoons, Raw

Banana – 2, ripe, small pieces

Directions:

Preheat the oven at 400F. Take a baking tray and line it with baking sheet. In a bowl, combine almonds, salt, vanilla and oats. In another small ball, combine honey, coconut oil (at room temperature), and bananas. Mash the bananas to make a smooth mixture. Now, add this banana mixture to the former dry mixture, combine until all ingredients coat each other well. Spread this mixture, granola, on the baking tray evenly. Place the tray into the preheated oven and bake it for at least 20 minutes. Check at 10 minutes interval, turn the granola upside down with the help of a spoon. Cool it down and store in a container for later use

Nutrition: Calories: 110 kcal; Fat: 5.4g; Carbohydrates: 14.2g; Sodium: 10.6mg; Protein: 2.9g

Chapter 2:Soups, Salads, and Sides

20. Spinach Soup with Dill and Basil

Preparation time: 10 minutes

Cooking time: 25 minutes

Servings: 8

Ingredients:

1 pound peeled and diced potatoes

1 tablespoon minced garlic

1 teaspoon dry mustard

6 cups vegetable broth

20 ounces chopped frozen spinach

2 cups chopped onion

1 ½ tablespoons salt

½ cup minced dill

1 cup basil

½ teaspoon ground black pepper

Directions:

Whisk onion, garlic, potatoes, broth, mustard, and salt in a pand

cook it over medium flame. When it starts boiling, low down the heat

and cover it with the lid and cook for 20 minutes. Add the remaining ingredients in it and blend it and cook it for few more minutes and serve it.

Nutrition: Carbohydrates 12g, protein 13g, fats 1g, calories 165.

21. Coconut Watercress Soup

Preparation time: 10 minutes

Cooking time: 20 minutes

Servings: 4

Ingredients:

1 teaspoon coconut oil

1 onion, diced

¾ cup coconut milk

Directions:

Preparing the ingredients.

Melt the coconut oil in a large pot over medium-high heat. Add the onion and cook until soft, about 5 minutes, then add the peas and the water. Bring to a boil, then lower the heat and add the watercress, mint, salt, and pepper.

Cover and simmer for 5 minutes. Stir in the coconut milk, and purée the soup until smooth in a blender or with an immersion blender. Try this soup with any other fresh, leafy green—anything from spinach to collard greens to arugula to swiss chard.

Nutrition: calories: 178; protein: 6g; total fat: 10g; carbohydrates: 18g; fiber: 5g

22. Roasted Red Pepper and Butternut Squash Soup

Preparation time: 10 minutes

Cooking time: 45 minutes

Servings: 6

Ingredients:

1 small butternut squash

1 tablespoon olive oil

1 teaspoon sea salt

2 red bell peppers

1 yellow onion

1 head garlic

2 cups water, or vegetable broth

Zest and juice of 1 lime

1 to 2 tablespoons tahini

Pinch cayenne pepper

½ teaspoon ground coriander

½ teaspoon ground cumin

Toasted squash seeds (optional)

Directions:

Preparing the ingredients.

Preheat the oven to 350°f.

Prepare the squash for roasting by cutting it in half lengthwise, scooping out the seeds, and poking some holes in the flesh with a fork. Reserve the seeds if desired.

Rub a small amount of oil over the flesh and skin, then rub with a bit of sea salt and put the halves skin-side down in a large baking dish. Put it in the oven while you prepare the rest of the vegetables.

Prepare the peppers the exact same way, except they do not need to be poked.

Slice the onion in half and rub oil on the exposed faces. Slice the top off the head of garlic and rub oil on the exposed flesh.

After the squash has cooked for 20 minutes, add the peppers, onion, and garlic, and roast for another 20 minutes. Optionally, you can toast the squash seeds by putting them in the oven in a separate baking dish 10 to 15 minutes before the vegetables are finished. Keep a close eye on them. When the vegetables are cooked, take them out and let them cool before handling them. The squash will be very soft when poked with a fork.

Scoop the flesh out of the squash skin into a large pot (if you have an immersion blender) or into a blender.

Chop the pepper roughly, remove the onion skin and chop the onion roughly, and squeeze the garlic cloves out of the head, all into the pot or blender. Add the water, the lime zest and juice, and the tahini. Purée the soup, adding more water if you like, to your desired consistency. Season with the salt, cayenne, coriander, and cumin. Serve garnished with toasted squash seeds (if using).

Nutrition: calories: 156; protein: 4g; total fat: 7g; saturated fat: 11g; carbohydrates: 22g; fiber: 5g

23. Tomato Pumpkin Soup

Preparation time: 25 minutes

Cooking time: 15 minutes

Servings: 4

Ingredients:

2 cups pumpkin, diced

1/2 cup tomato, chopped

1/2 cup onion, chopped

1 1/2 tsp curry powder

1/2 tsp paprika

2 cups vegetable stock

1 tsp olive oil

1/2 tsp garlic, minced

Directions:

In a saucepan, add oil, garlic, and onion and sauté for 3 minutes over medium heat.

Add remaining ingredients into the saucepan and bring to boil.

Reduce heat and cover and simmer for 10 minutes.

Puree the soup using a blender until smooth.

Stir well and serve warm.

Nutrition: calories 70; fat 2.7 g; carbohydrates 13.8 g; sugar 6.3 g;

protein 1.9 g; cholesterol 0 mg

24. Cauliflower Spinach Soup

Preparation time: 45 minutes

Cooking time: 25 minutes

Servings: 5

Ingredients:

1/2 cup unsweetened coconut milk

5 oz fresh spinach, chopped

5 watercress, chopped

8 cups vegetable stock

1 lb cauliflower, chopped

Salt

Directions:

Add stock and cauliflower in a large saucepan and bring to boil over medium heat for 15 minutes.

Add spinach and watercress and cook for another 10 minutes.

Remove from heat and puree the soup using a blender until smooth.

Add coconut milk and stir well. Season with salt.

Stir well and serve hot.

Nutrition: calories 153; fat 8.3 g; carbohydrates 8.7 g; sugar 4.3 g; protein 11.9 g; cholesterol 0 mg

25. Avocado Mint Soup

Preparation time: 10 minutes

Cooking time: 10 minutes

Servings: 2

Ingredients:

1 medium avocado, peeled, pitted, and cut into pieces

1 cup coconut milk

2 romaine lettuce leaves

20 fresh mint leaves

1 tbsp fresh lime juice

1/8 tsp salt

Directions:

Add all ingredients into the blender and blend until smooth. Soup should be thick not as a puree.

Pour into the serving bowls and place in the refrigerator for 10 minutes.

Stir well and serve chilled.

Nutrition: calories 268; fat 25.6 g; carbohydrates 10.2 g; sugar 0.6 g; protein 2.7 g; cholesterol 0 mg

26. Creamy Squash Soup

Preparation time: 35 minutes

Cooking time: 22 minutes

Servings: 8

Ingredients:

3 cups butternut squash, chopped

1 ½ cups unsweetened coconut milk

1 tbsp coconut oil

1 tsp dried onion flakes

1 tbsp curry powder

4 cups water

1 garlic clove

1 tsp kosher salt

Directions:

Add squash, coconut oil, onion flakes, curry powder, water, garlic, and salt into a large saucepan. Bring to boil over high heat.

Turn heat to medium and simmer for 20 minutes.

Puree the soup using a blender until smooth. Return soup to the saucepan and stir in coconut milk and cook for 2 minutes.

Stir well and serve hot.

Nutrition: calories 146; fat 12.6 g; carbohydrates 9.4 g; sugar 2.8 g;

protein 1.7 g; cholesterol 0 mg

27. Cucumber Edamame Salad

Preparation time: 5 minutes

Cooking time: 8 minutes

Servings: 2

Ingredients:

3 tbsp. Avocado oil

1 cup cucumber, sliced into thin rounds

½ cup fresh sugar snap peas, sliced or whole

½ cup fresh edamame

¼ cup radish, sliced

1 large avocado, peeled, pitted, sliced

1 nori sheet, crumbled

2 tsp. Roasted sesame seeds

1 tsp. Salt

Directions:

Bring a medium-sized pot filled halfway with water to a boil over medium-high heat.

Add the sugar snaps and cook them for about 2 minutes.

Take the pot off the heat, drain the excess water, transfer the sugar snaps to a medium-sized bowl and set aside for now.

Fill the pot with water again, add the teaspoon of salt and bring to a boil over medium-high heat.

Add the edamame to the pot and let them cook for about 6 minutes.

Take the pot off the heat, drain the excess water, transfer the
soybeans to the bowl with sugar snaps and let them cool down for
about 5 minutes.

Combine all ingredients, except the nori crumbs and roasted sesame
seeds, in a medium-sized bowl.

Carefully stir, using a spoon, until all ingredients are evenly coated in
oil.

Top the salad with the nori crumbs and roasted sesame seeds.

Transfer the bowl to the fridge and allow the salad to cool for at least
30 minutes.

Serve chilled and enjoy!

Nutrition: Calories 409 Carbohydrates 7.1 g Fats 38.25 g
Protein 7.6g

28. Best Broccoli Salad

Preparation time: 15 minutes

Chilling time: 1 hour

Servings: 8

Ingredients:

8 cups diced broccoli

¼ cup sunflower seeds

3 tablespoons apple cider vinegar

½ cup dried cranberries

1/3 cup cubed onion

1 cup mayonnaise

½ cup bacon bits

2 tablespoons sugar

½ teaspoon salt and ground black pepper

Directions:

In a bowl, mix vinegar, salt, pepper, mayonnaise, and sugar. Mix it well. In another bowl, mix all the remaining ingredients and pour the prepared mayonnaise dressing and mix it well. Before serving to refrigerate it for at least an hour.

Nutrition: Carbohydrates 17g, protein 6g, fats 26g, calories 317

29. Rainbow Orzo Salad

Preparation time: 10 minutes

Cooking time: 20 minutes

Servings: 1

Ingredients:

1 chopped onion

25g grated feta cheese

2 sliced bell peppers

1 tablespoon olive oil

6 sliced tomatoes

2 tablespoons chopped basil

25g orzo pasta

Directions:

Preheat the oven at 350f temperature. Prepare a baking sheet and place the onion and bell peppers and drizzle half olive oil. Bake it for around 15 minutes. Add tomatoes on it and bake for an additional 5 minutes. Meanwhile, cook the orzo according to the given directions on the pack and cool it. Now toss it with the baked vegetables and top it with cheese, basil and remaining oil and serve it.

Nutrition: Carbohydrates 52g, protein 13g, fats 18g, calories 422, sugar 30g.

30. Broccoli Pasta Salad

Preparation time: 15 minutes

Chilling time: 30 minutes

Servings: 12

Ingredients:

1-pound cooked pasta

2 diced broccoli florets

1 chopped onion

1 cup grated cheese

12 ounce cooked and finely chopped bacon

¾ teaspoon salt

¾ teaspoon ground black pepper

1 cup mayonnaise

Directions:

Take a bowl and mix all the ingredients until all of them combined well. Cover it with the plastic wrap and place it in the refrigerator for at least 30 minutes and serve it. You can keep it in the refrigerator for 3 days.

Nutrition: Carbohydrates 36g, protein 14g, fats 29g, calories 461.

31. Eggplant & Roasted Tomato Farro Salad

Preparation time: 1 hour

Cooking time: 1 hour 30 minutes

Servings: 3

Ingredients:

4 small eggplants

1 ½ cups chopped cherry tomatoes

¾ cup uncooked faro

1 tablespoon olive oil

1 minced garlic clove

½ cup rinsed and drained chickpeas

1 tablespoon basil

1 tablespoon arugula

½ teaspoon salt and ground black pepper

1 tablespoon vinegar

½ cup toasted pine nuts

Directions:

Preheat the oven at 300f temperature and prepare a baking sheet.

Place cherry tomatoes on the baking liner and drizzle olive oil, salt, and black pepper on it and bake it for 30 to 35 minutes. Cook the faro in the salted water for 30 to 40 minutes. Slice the eggplant and salt it and leave it for 30 minutes. After that, rinse it with water and dry it kitchen towel. Now peeled and sliced the eggplants. Now place these slices on the baking liner and season it with salt, pepper and olive oil. Bake it for 15 to 20 minutes in the preheated oven at the 450f temperature. Flip the sides of eggplant and bake it for an additional 15 to 20 minutes. Bake the pine nuts for 5 minutes and sauté the garlic. Now mix all the ingredients in a bowl and serve it.

Nutrition: Carbohydrates 37g, protein 9g, fats 25g, calories 399.

32. Garden Patch Sandwiches on Multigrain Bread

Preparation time: 15 minutes

Cooking time: 0 minutes

Servings: 4 sandwiches

Ingredients:

1pound extra-firm tofu, drained and patted dry

1 medium red bell pepper, finely chopped

1 celery rib, finely chopped

3 green onions, minced

$1/$ cup shelled sunflower seeds

$1/$ cup vegan mayonnaise, homemade or store-bought

$1/$ teaspoon salt

$1/$ teaspoon celery salt

$1/$ teaspoon freshly ground black pepper

8 slices whole grain bread

4 ($1/$ -inch) slices ripe tomato

4 lettuce leaves

Directions:

Crumble the tofu and place it in a large bowl. Add the bell pepper,

celery, green onions, and sunflower seeds. Stir in the mayonnaise, salt, celery salt, and pepper and mix until well combined.

Toast the bread, if desired. Spread the mixture evenly onto 4 slices

of the bread. Top each with a tomato slice, lettuce leaf, and the

remaining bread. Cut the sandwiches diagonally in half and serve.

33. Garden Salad Wraps

Preparation time: 15 minutes

Cooking time: 10 minutes

Servings: 4 wraps

Ingredients:

6 tablespoons olive oil

1-pound extra-firm tofu, drained, patted dry, and cut into $\frac{1}{}$ -inch strips

1 tablespoon soy sauce

$\frac{1}{}$ cup apple cider vinegar

1 teaspoon yellow or spicy brown mustard

$\frac{1}{}$ teaspoon salt

$\frac{1}{}$ teaspoon freshly ground black pepper

3 cups shredded romaine lettuce

3 ripe roma tomatoes, finely chopped

1 large carrot, shredded

1 medium english cucumber, peeled and chopped

$\frac{1}{}$ cup minced red onion

$\frac{1}{}$ cup sliced pitted green olives

4 (10-inch) whole-grain flour tortillas or lavash flatbread

Directions:

In a large skillet, heat 2 tablespoons of the oil over medium heat.

Add the tofu and cook until golden brown, about 10 minutes. Sprinkle

with soy sauce and set aside to cool.

In a small bowl, combine the vinegar, mustard, salt, and pepper with

the remaining 4 tablespoons oil, stirring to blend well. Set aside.

In a large bowl, combine the lettuce, tomatoes, carrot, cucumber,

onion, and olives. Pour on the dressing and toss to coat.

To assemble wraps, place 1 tortilla on a work surface and spread

with about one-quarter of the salad. Place a few strips of tofu on the

tortilla and roll up tightly. Slice in half

34. Marinated Mushroom Wraps

Preparation time: 15 minutes

Cooking time: 0 minutes

Servings: 2 wraps

Ingredients:

3 tablespoons soy sauce

3 tablespoons fresh lemon juice

1½ tablespoons toasted sesame oil

2 portobello mushroom caps, cut into ¼-inch strips

1 ripe hass avocado, pitted and peeled

2 cups fresh baby spinach leaves

1 medium red bell pepper, cut into ¼-inch strips

1 ripe tomato, chopped

Salt and freshly ground black pepper

Directions:

In a medium bowl, combine the soy sauce, 2 tablespoons of the lemon juice, and the oil. Add the portobello strips, toss to combine, and marinate for 1 hour or overnight. Drain the mushrooms and set aside.

Mash the avocado with the remaining 1 tablespoon of lemon juice.

To assemble wraps, place 1 tortilla on a work surface and spread with some of the mashed avocado. Top with a layer of baby spinach leaves. In the lower third of each tortilla, arrange strips of the soaked mushrooms and some of the bell pepper strips. Sprinkle with the tomato and salt and black pepper to taste. Roll up tightly and cut in half diagonally. Repeat with the remaining ingredients and serve.

35. Tamari Toasted Almonds

Preparation time: 2 minutes

Cooking time: 8 minutes

Servings: ½ cup

Ingredients:

½ cup raw almonds, or sunflower seeds

2 tablespoons tamari, or soy sauce

1 teaspoon toasted sesame oil

Directions:

Preparing the ingredients.

Heat a dry skillet to medium-high heat, then add the almonds, stirring very frequently to keep them from burning. Once the almonds are toasted, 7 to 8 minutes for almonds, or 3 to 4 minutes for sunflower seeds, pour the tamari and sesame oil into the hot skillet and stir to coat.

You can turn off the heat, and as the almonds cool the tamari mixture will stick to and dry on the nuts.

Nutrition: calories: 89; total fat: 8g; carbs: 3g; fiber: 2g; protein: 4g

36. Nourishing Whole-Grain Porridge

Preparation time: 2 hours and 10 minutes

Cooking time: 2 hours

Servings: 4

Ingredients:

3/4 cup of steel-cut oats, rinsed and soaked overnight

3/4 cup of whole barley, rinsed and soaked overnight

1/2 cup of cornmeal

1 teaspoon of salt

3 tablespoons of brown sugar

1 cinnamon stick, about 3 inches long

1 teaspoon of vanilla extract, unsweetened

4 1/2 cups of water

Directions:

Using a 6-quarts slow cooker, place all the ingredients and stir properly.

Cover it with the lid, plug in the slow cooker and let it cook for 2 hours or until grains get soft, while stirring halfway through.

Serve the porridge with fruits.

Nutrition: Calories: 129 Cal, Carbohydrates:22g, Protein:5g, Fats:2g, Fiber:4g.

37. Pungent Mushroom Barley Risotto

Preparation time: 3 hours and 30 minutes

Cooking time: 3 hours and 9 minutes

Servings: 4

Ingredients:

1 1/2 cups of hulled barley, rinsed and soaked overnight

8 ounces of carrots, peeled and chopped

1 pound of mushrooms, sliced

1 large white onion, peeled and chopped

3/4 teaspoon of salt

1/2 teaspoon of ground black pepper

4 sprigs thyme

1/4 cup of chopped parsley

2/3 cup of grated vegan Parmesan cheese

1 tablespoon of apple cider vinegar

2 tablespoons of olive oil

1 1/2 cups of vegetable broth

Directions:

Place a large non-stick skillet pan over a medium-high heat, add the oil and let it heat until it gets hot.

Add the onion along with 1/4 teaspoon of each the salt and black pepper.

Cook it for 5 minutes or until it turns golden brown.

Then add the mushrooms and continue cooking for 2 minutes.

Add the barley, thyme and cook for another 2 minutes.

Transfer this mixture to a 6-quarts slow cooker and add the carrots, 1/4 teaspoon of salt, and the vegetable broth.

Stir properly and cover it with the lid.

Plug in the slow cooker, let it cook for 3 hours at the high heat setting or until the grains absorb all the cooking liquid and the vegetables get soft.

Remove the thyme sprigs, pour in the remaining ingredients except for parsley and stir properly.

Pour in the warm water and stir properly until the risotto reaches your desired state.

Add the seasoning, then garnish it with parsley and serve.

Nutrition: Calories:321 Cal, Carbohydrates:48g, Protein:12g, Fats:10g, Fiber:11g.

Chapter 3 :Entrées

38. Black Bean Dip

Preparation time: 1 hour and 30 minutes

Cooking time: 1 hour

Servings: 10

Ingredients:

2 15-ounce cans black beans, rinsed and drained

1 jalapeno pepper, seeded and minced

½ of a red bell pepper, seeded and diced

½ of a yellow bell pepper, seeded and diced

½ of s small red onion, diced

1 cup fresh cilantro, finely chopped

Zest of 1 lime

Juice of 1 lime

1 10-ounce can Ro*tel, drained

½ teaspoon Kosher salt

¼ teaspoon ground black pepper

Directions:

In a large bowl, combine the garlic, green onions, beans, jalapeno,

red and yellow bell pepper, onion, cilantro and mix together well.

Add the lime zest and juice, Ro-tel, salt and pepper and mix. Adjust seasoning to your own taste.

Refrigerate for at one hour, minimum, before serving, so the flavors have time to blend. Serve with wheat tortilla slices that have been crisped in the oven or with wheat or sesame crackers.

39. Cannellini Bean Cashew Dip

Preparation time: 1 hour

Cooking time: 1 hour

Servings: 8

Ingredients:

1 15-ounce can cannellini beans, rinsed and drained

½ cup raw cashews

1 clove garlic, smashed

2 tablespoons diced, red bell pepper

½ teaspoon sea salt

¼ teaspoon cayenne pepper

4 teaspoons lemon juice

2 tablespoons water

Dill sprigs or weed for garnish

Directions:

Place the beans, cashews, garlic and bell pepper in the food

processor and pulse several times to break it up.

Add the salt, cayenne, lemon juice and water and process until

smooth.Scrape into a bowl, cover and refrigerate for at least an hour beforeserving.Garnish with fresh dill and serve with vegetables, crackers or pita

chips.

40. Cauliflower Popcorn

Preparation time: 1 day and 1 hour

Cooking time: 1 day

Servings: 2

Ingredients:

¼ cup sun-dried tomatoes

¾ cup dates

2 heads cauliflower

½ cup water

2 tablespoons raw tahini

1 tablespoon apple cider vinegar

2 teaspoons onion powder

2 teaspoons garlic powder

1 teaspoon ground cayenne pepper

2 tablespoons nutritional yeast (optional)

Directions:

Cover the sun-dried tomatoes warm water and let them soak for an hour.

If the dates are not soft and fresh, soak them in warm water for an hour in another bowl.

Cut the cauliflower in very small, bite-sized pieces then set aside.

Put the drained tomatoes and dates in a blender along with the water, tahini, apple cider vinegar, onion powder, garlic powder, cayenne pepper, nutritional yeast and turmeric. Blend into a thick, smooth consistency.

Pour this mixture into the bowl, atop the cauliflower and mix so that all the pieces are coated.

Place the cauliflower in the dehydrator and spread it out to make a single layer. Sprinkle with a little sea salt and set for 115 degrees, Fahrenheit for 12 to 24 hours or until it becomes exactly as crunchy as you like it. I let mine go for 15 to 16 hours, but the time will vary based on your taste preference as well as the ambient humidity. Store in an airtight container until serving.

41. Cinnamon Apple Chips with Dip

Preparation time: 3 hours and 30 minutes

Cooking time: 3 hours

Servings: 2

Ingredients:

1 cup raw cashews

2 apples, thinly sliced

1 lemon

1½ cups water, divided

Cinnamon plus more to dust the chips

Another medium cored apple quartered

1 tablespoon honey or agave

1 teaspoon cinnamon

¼ teaspoon sea salt

Directions:

Place the cashews in a bowl of warm water, deep enough to cover them and let them soak overnight.

Preheat the oven to 200 degrees, Fahrenheit. Line two baking sheets with parchment paper.

Juice the lemon into a large glass bowl and add two cups of the water. Place the sliced apples in the water as you cut them and when done, swish them around and drain.

Spread the apple slices across the baking sheet in a single layer and sprinkle with a little cinnamon. Bake for 90 minutes.

Remove the slices from the oven and flip each of them over. Put them back in the oven and bake for another 90 minutes, or until they are crisp. Remember, they will get crisper as they cool.

While the apple slices are cooking, drain the cashews and put them in a blender, along with the quartered apple, the honey, a teaspoon of cinnamon and a half cup of the remaining water. Process until thick and creamy. I like to refrigerate my dip for about an hour to chill, before serve alongside the room temperature apple slices.

42. Crunchy Asparagus Spears

Preparation time: 25 minutes

Cooking time: 25 minutes

Servings: 4

Ingredients:

1 bunch asparagus spears (about 12 spears)

¼ cup nutritional yeast

2 tablespoons hemp seeds

1 teaspoon garlic powder

¼ teaspoon paprika (or more if you like paprika)

⅛ teaspoon ground pepper

¼ cup whole-wheat breadcrumbs

Juice of ½ lemon

Directions:

Preheat the oven to 350 degrees, Fahrenheit. Line a baking sheet with parchment paper.

Wash the asparagus, snapping off the white part at the bottom. Save it for making vegetable stock.

Mix together the nutritional yeast, hemp seed, garlic powder, paprika, pepper and breadcrumbs.

Place asparagus spears on the baking sheets giving them a little room in between and sprinkle with the mixture in the bowl.

Bake for up to 25 minutes, until crispy.

Serve with lemon juice if desired.

43. Cucumber Bites with Chive and Sunflower Seeds

Preparation time: 5 minutes

Cooking time: 5 minutes

Servings: 2

Ingredients:

1 cup raw sunflower seed

½ teaspoon salt

½ cup chopped fresh chives

1 clove garlic, chopped

2 tablespoons red onion, minced

2 tablespoons lemon juice

½ cup water (might need more or less)

4 large cucumbers

Directions:

Place the sunflower seeds and salt in the food processor and process to a fine powder. It will take only about 10 seconds.

Add the chives, garlic, onion, lemon juice and water and process until creamy, scraping down the sides frequently. The mixture should be very creamy; if not, add a little more water.

Cut the cucumbers into 1½-inch coin-like pieces.

Spread a spoonful of the sunflower mixture on top and set on a platter. Sprinkle more chopped chives on top and refrigerate until ready to serve.

44. Garlicky Kale Chips

Preparation time: 1 hour and 30 min

Cooking time: 1 hour

Servings: 2

Ingredients:

4 cloves garlic

1 cup olive oil

8 to 10 cups fresh kale, chopped

1 tablespoon of garlic-flavored olive oil

½ teaspoon garlic salt

½ teaspoon pepper

1 pinch red pepper flakes (optional)

Directions:

Peel and crush the garlic clove and place it in a small jar with a lid. Pour the olive oil over the top, cover tightly and shake. This will keep in the refrigerator for several days. When you're ready to use it, strain out the garlic and retain the oil.

Preheat the oven to 175 degrees, Fahrenheit.

Spread out the kale on a baking sheet and drizzle with the olive oil.

Sprinkle with garlic salt, pepper and red pepper flakes.

Bake for an hour, remove from the oven and let the chips cool.

Store in an airtight container if you don't plan to eat them right away.

45. Hummus-stuffed Baby Potatoes

Preparation time: 30 minutes

Cooking time: 30 minutes

Servings: 2

Ingredients:

12 small red potatoes, walnut-sized or slightly larger

Hummus

2 green onions, thinly sliced

¼ teaspoon paprika, for garnish

Directions:

Place two to three inches of water in a saucepan, set a steamer

inside and bring the water to a boil.

Place the whole potatoes in the steamer basket and steam for about

20 minutes or until soft. Keep the pan from boiling dry by adding

additional hot water as needed.Dump the potatoes into a colander and run cold water over them until they can be handled.

Cut each potato open and scoop out most of the pulp, leaving the

skin and a thin layer of potato intact. Mix the hummus with most of the green onions (keep enough for garnish) and spoon a little into the area where the potato has been scooped out.

Sprinkle each filled potato half with paprika and serve.

46. Homemade Trail Mix

Preparation time: 20 minutes

Cooking time: 20 minutes

Servings: 2

Ingredients:

½ cup uncooked old-fashioned oatmeal

½ cup chopped dates

2 cups whole grain cereal

¼ cup raisins

¼ cup almonds

¼ cup walnuts

Directions:

Mix all the ingredients in a large bowl.

Place in an airtight container until ready to use.

47. Nut Butter Maple Dip

Preparation time: 1 hour

Cooking time: 1 hour

Servings:

Ingredients:

½ tablespoon ground flaxseed

1 teaspoon ground cinnamon

½ tablespoon maple syrup

2 tablespoons cashew milk

¾ cups crunchy, unsweetened peanut butter

Directions:

In a bowl, combine the flaxseed, cinnamon, maple syrup, cashew milk and peanut butter.

Use a fork to mix everything in. I stir it like I'm scrambling eggs. The mixture should be creamy. If it's too runny, add a little more peanut butter; if it's too thick, add a little more cashew milk.

Refrigerate for about an hour, covered and serve.

48. Oven Baked Sesame Fries

Preparation time: 30 minutes

Cooking time: 30 minutes

Servings: 4

Ingredients:

1 pound Yukon Gold potatoes, skins on and cut into wedges

2 tablespoons sesame seeds

1 tablespoon potato starch

1 tablespoon sesame oil

Salt to taste

Black pepper to taste

Directions:

Preheat the oven to 425 degrees, Fahrenheit and cover a baking

sheet or two with parchment paper.

Cut the potatoes and place in a large bowl.

Add the sesame seeds, potato starch, sesame oil, salt and pepper.

Toss with your hands and make sure all the wedges are coated. Add

more sesame seeds or oil if needed.Spread the potato wedges on the
baking sheets with some room between each wedge.

Bake for 15 minutes, flip the wedges over and then return them to

the oven for 10 to 15 more minutes, until they look golden and crispy.

49. Pumpkin Orange Spice Hummus

Preparation time: 30 minutes

Cooking time: 30 minutes

Servings: 3

Ingredients:

1 cup canned, unsweetened pumpkin puree

1 16-ounce can garbanzo beans, rinsed and drained

1 tablespoon apple cider vinegar

1 tablespoon maple syrup

¼ cup tahini

1 tablespoon fresh orange juice

½ teaspoon orange zest and additional zest for garnish

⅛ teaspoon ground cinnamon

⅛ teaspoon ground ginger

⅛ teaspoon ground nutmeg

¼ teaspoon salt

Directions:

Pour the pumpkin puree and garbanzo beans into a food processor and pulse to break up.

Add the vinegar, syrup, tahini, orange juice and orange zest pulse a few times.

Add the cinnamon, ginger, nutmeg and salt and process until smooth and creamy.

Serve in a bowl sprinkled with more orange zest with wheat crackers alongside.

50. Quick English Muffin Mexican Pizzas

Preparation time: 30 minutes

Cooking time: 15 minutes

Servings:

Ingredients:

2 whole-wheat English muffins separated

⅓ cup tomato salsa

¼ cup refried beans

1 small jalapeno, seeded and sliced

¼ cup onion, sliced

2 tablespoons diced plum or cherry tomato

⅓ cup vegan cheese shreds (pepper jack is really tasty!)

Directions:

Preheat the oven to 400 degrees, Fahrenheit and cover a baking sheet with foil. The foil makes the crust crispier.

Separate the English muffin and spread on some salsa and refried beans.Place some of the jalapenos and onions on top and sprinkle the cheese over all.

Place on the baking sheet and bake for 10 to 15 minutes or until brown. You can turn on the broiler for a minute or two to melt the cheese.

51. Quinoa Trail Mix Cups

Preparation time: 30 minutes

Cooking time: 30 minutes

Servings: 16

Ingredients:

2 tablespoons ground flaxseed

⅓ cup unsweetened soy milk

1 cup old-fashioned rolled oats

1 cup cooked and cooled quinoa

¼ cup brown sugar

1 teaspoon ground cinnamon

¼ teaspoon salt

¼ cup pumpkin or sunflower seeds

¼ cup shredded coconut

½ cup almonds

½ cup raisins or dried cherries/cranberries

Directions:

Whisk the flaxseed and milk together in a small bowl and set aside for 10 minutes so the seed can absorb the milk.

Preheat the oven to 350 degrees, Fahrenheit and coat a muffin tin with coconut oil.

In a large bowl, mix the oats, quinoa, brown sugar, cinnamon, salt, pumpkin seeds, coconut, almonds and raisins.

Stir in the flaxseed and milk mixture and combine thoroughly.

Place two heaping teaspoons of the trail mix mixture in each muffin cup. When done, wet your fingers and press down on each muffin cup to compact the trail mix.

Bake for 12 minutes.

Cool completely before removing and each little cup will fall out.

Store in an airtight container.

Chapter 4 : Smoothies and Beverages

52. Fruity Smoothie

Preparation Time: 10 Minutes

Cooking time: 0 minute

Servings: 1

Ingredients:

¾ cup soy yogurt

½ cup pineapple juice

1 cup pineapple chunks

1 cup raspberries, sliced

1 cup blueberries, sliced

Direction:

Process the ingredients in a blender.

Chill before serving.

Nutrition: Calories 279, Total Fat 2 g, Saturated Fat 0 g Cholesterol 4 mg, Sodium 149 mg, Total Carbohydrate 56 g Dietary Fiber 7 g, Protein 12 g, Total Sugars 46 g Potassium 719 mg

53. Energizing Ginger Detox Tonic

Preparation time: 15 minutes

Cooking time: 10 minutes

Servings: 2

Ingredients:

1/2 teaspoon of grated ginger, fresh

1 small lemon slice

1/8 teaspoon of cayenne pepper

1/8 teaspoon of ground turmeric

1/8 teaspoon of ground cinnamon

1 teaspoon of maple syrup

1 teaspoon of apple cider vinegar

2 cups of boiling water

Directions:

Pour the boiling water into a small saucepan, add and stir the ginger,

then let it rest for 8 to 10 minutes, before covering the pan.Pass the mixture through a strainer and into the liquid, add the

cayenne pepper, turmeric, cinnamon and stir properly.Add the maple syrup, vinegar, and lemon slice.Add and stir an infused lemon and serve immediately.

Nutrition: Calories:80 Cal, Carbohydrates:0g, Protein:0g, Fats:0g,

Fiber:0g.

54. Warm Spiced Lemon Drink

Preparation time: 2 hours and 10 minutes

Cooking time: 2 hours

Servings: 12

Ingredients:

1 cinnamon stick, about 3 inches long

1/2 teaspoon of whole cloves

2 cups of coconut sugar

4 fluid of ounce pineapple juice

1/2 cup and 2 tablespoons of lemon juice

12 fluid ounce of orange juice

2 1/2 quarts of water

Directions:

Pour water into a 6-quarts slow cooker and stir the sugar and lemon juice properly.

Wrap the cinnamon, the whole cloves in cheesecloth and tie its corners with string.

Immerse this cheesecloth bag in the liquid present in the slow cooker and cover it with the lid.

Then plug in the slow cooker and let it cook on high heat setting for 2 hours or until it is heated thoroughly.

When done, discard the cheesecloth bag and serve the drink hot or cold.

Nutrition: Calories:15 Cal, Carbohydrates:3.2g, Protein:0.1g, Fats:0g, Fiber:0g.

55. Soothing Ginger Tea Drink

Preparation time: 2 hours and 15 minutes

Cooking time: 2 hours and 10 minutes

Servings: 8

Ingredients:

1 tablespoon of minced ginger root

2 tablespoons of honey

15 green tea bags

32 fluid ounce of white grape juice

2 quarts of boiling water

Directions:

Pour water into a 4-quarts slow cooker, immerse tea bags, cover the cooker and let stand for 10 minutes.

After 10 minutes, remove and discard tea bags and stir in remaining

ingredients. Return cover to slow cooker, then plug in and let cook at high heat setting for 2 hours or until heated through.

When done, strain the liquid and serve hot or cold.

Nutrition: Calories:45 Cal, Carbohydrates:12g, Protein:0g, Fats:0g, Fiber:0g.

56. Nice Spiced Cherry Cider

Preparation time: 4 hours and 5 minutes

Cooking time: 4 hours

Servings: 16

Ingredients:

2 cinnamon sticks, each about 3 inches long

6-ounce of cherry gelatin

4 quarts of apple cider

Directions:

Using a 6-quarts slow cooker, pour the apple cider and add the cinnamon stick.

Stir, then cover the slow cooker with its lid. Plug in the cooker and let it cook for 3 hours at the high heat setting or until it is heated thoroughly.

Then add and stir the gelatin properly, then continue cooking for another hour.

When done, remove the cinnamon sticks and serve the drink hot or cold.

Nutrition: , Calories:100 Cal, Carbohydrates:0g, Protein:0g, Fats:0g, Fiber:0g.

57. Fragrant Spiced Coffee

Preparation time: 3 hours and 10 minutes

Cooking time: 3 hours

Servings: 8

Ingredients:

4 cinnamon sticks, each about 3 inches long

1 1/2 teaspoons of whole cloves

1/3 cup of honey

2-ounce of chocolate syrup

1/2 teaspoon of anise extract

8 cups of brewed coffee

Directions:

Pour the coffee in a 4-quarts slow cooker and pour in the remaining

ingredients except for cinnamon and stir properly.

Wrap the whole cloves in cheesecloth and tie its corners with

strings.Immerse this cheesecloth bag in the liquid present in the slow cookerand cover it with the lid.Then plug in the slow cooker and let it cook on the low heat setting

for 3 hours or until heated thoroughly.

When done, discard the cheesecloth bag and serve.

Nutrition: Calories:150 Cal, Carbohydrates:35g, Protein:3g, Fats:0g,

Fiber:0g.

58. Tangy Spiced Cranberry Drink

Preparation time: 3 hours and 10 minutes

Cooking time: 3 hours

Servings: 14

Ingredients:

1 1/2 cups of coconut sugar

12 whole cloves

2 fluid ounce of lemon juice

6 fluid ounce of orange juice

32 fluid ounce of cranberry juice

8 cups of hot water

1/2 cup of Red Hot candies

Directions:

Pour the water into a 6-quarts slow cooker along with the cranberry juice, orange juice, and the lemon juice.

Stir the sugar properly.

Wrap the whole cloves in a cheese cloth, tie its corners with strings, and immerse it in the liquid present inside the slow cooker.

Add the red hot candies to the slow cooker and cover it with the lid.

Then plug in the slow cooker and let it cook on the low heat setting for 3 hours or until it is heated thoroughly.

When done, discard the cheesecloth bag and serve.

Nutrition: Calories:89 Cal, Carbohydrates:27g, Protein:0g, Fats:0g, Fiber:1g.

59. Warm Pomegranate Punch

Preparation time: 3 hours and 15 minutes

Cooking time: 3 hours

Servings: 10

Ingredients:

3 cinnamon sticks, each about 3 inches long

12 whole cloves

1/2 cup of coconut sugar

1/3 cup of lemon juice

32 fluid ounce of pomegranate juice

32 fluid ounce of apple juice, unsweetened

16 fluid ounce of brewed tea

Directions:

Using a 4-quart slow cooker, pour the lemon juice, pomegranate, juice apple juice, tea, and then sugar.

Wrap the whole cloves and cinnamon stick in a cheese cloth, tie its corners with a string, and immerse it in the liquid present in the slow cooker.Then cover it with the lid, plug in the slow cooker and let it cook atthe low heat setting for 3 hours or until it is heated thoroughly.When done, discard the cheesecloth bag and serve it hot or cold.Nutrition: Calories:253 Cal, Carbohydrates:58g, Protein:7g, Fats:2g,Fiber:3g.

60. Rich Truffle Hot Chocolate

Preparation time: 2 hours and 10 minutes

Cooking time: 2 hours

Servings: 4

Ingredients:

1/3 cup of cocoa powder, unsweetened

1/3 cup of coconut sugar

1/8 teaspoon of salt

1/8 teaspoon of ground cinnamon

1 teaspoon of vanilla extract, unsweetened

32 fluid ounce of coconut milk

Directions:

Using a 2 quarts slow cooker, add all the ingredients and stir properly.

Cover it with the lid, then plug in the slow cooker and cook it for 2 hours on the high heat setting or until it is heated thoroughly.

When done, serve right away.

Nutrition: Calories:67 Cal, Carbohydrates:13g, Protein:2g, Fats:2g, Fiber:2.3g.

61. Ultimate Mulled Wine

Preparation time: 35 minutes

Cooking time: 30 minutes

Servings: 6

Ingredients:

1 cup of cranberries, fresh

2 oranges, juiced

1 tablespoon of whole cloves

2 cinnamon sticks, each about 3 inches long

1 tablespoon of star anise

1/3 cup of honey

8 fluid ounce of apple cider

8 fluid ounce of cranberry juice

24 fluid ounce of red wine

Directions:

Using a 4 quarts slow cooker, add all the ingredients and stir

properly.Cover it with the lid, then plug in the slow cooker and cook it for 30 minutes on thee high heat setting or until it gets warm thoroughly.When done, strain the wine and serve right away.

Nutrition: Calories:202 Cal, Carbohydrates:25g, Protein:0g, Fats:0g,

Fiber:0g.

62. Pleasant Lemonade

Preparation time: 3 hours and 15 minutes

Cooking time: 3 hours

Servings: 10 servings

Ingredients:

Cinnamon sticks for serving

2 cups of coconut sugar

1/4 cup of honey

3 cups of lemon juice. fresh

32 fluid ounce of water

Directions:

Using a 4-quarts slow cooker, place all the ingredients except for the cinnamon sticks and stir properly.

Cover it with the lid, then plug in the slow cooker and cook it for 3 hours on the low heat setting or until it is heated thoroughly.

When done, stir properly and serve with the cinnamon sticks.

Nutrition: Calories:146 Cal, Carbohydrates:34g, Protein:0g, Fats:0g, Fiber:0g.

63. Pineapple, Banana & Spinach Smoothie

Preparation Time: 10 Minutes

Cooking time: 0 minute

Servings: 1

Ingredients:

½ cup almond milk

¼ cup soy yogurt

1 cup spinach

1 cup banana

1 cup pineapple chunks

1 tbsp. chia seeds

Direction:

Add all the ingredients in a blender.

Blend until smooth.

Chill in the refrigerator before serving.

Nutrition: Calories 297, Total Fat 6 g, Saturated Fat 1 g, Cholesterol 4 mg Sodium 145 mg, Total Carbohydrate 54 g, Dietary Fiber 10 g Protein 13 g, Total Sugars 29g, Potassium 1038 mg

64. Kale & Avocado Smoothie

Preparation Time: 10 Minutes

Cooking time: 0 minute

Servings: 1

Ingredients:

1 ripe banana

1 cup kale

1 cup almond milk

¼ avocado

1 tbsp. chia seeds

2 tsp. honey

1 cup ice cubes

Direction:

Blend all the ingredients until smooth.

Nutrition: Calories 343 Total Fat 14 g Saturated Fat 2 g

Cholesterol 0 mg Sodium 199 mg Total Carbohydrate 55 g

Dietary Fiber 12 g Protein 6 g Total Sugars 29 g Potassium 1051

mg

65. Coconut & Strawberry Smoothie

Preparation Time: 10 Minutes

Cooking Time: 0 minutes

Serves: 1

Calories: 278

Protein: 14 Grams

Fat: 2 Grams

Carbs: 57 Grams

Ingredients:

1 Cup Strawberries, Frozen & Thawed Slightly

1 Ripe Banana, Sliced & Frozen

½ Cup Coconut Milk, Light

½ Cup Vegan Yogurt

1 Tablespoon Chia Seeds

1 Teaspoon Lime juice, Fresh

4 Ice Cubes

Directions:

Blend everything together until smooth, and serve immediately.

66. Pumpkin Chia Smoothie

Preparation Time: 5 Minutes

Cooking Time: 0 minutes

Serves: 1

Calories: 726

Protein: 5.5 Grams

Fat: 69.8 Grams

Carbs: 15 Grams

Ingredients:

3 Tablespoons Pumpkin Puree

1 Tablespoon MCT Oil

¾ Cup Coconut Milk, Full Fat

½ Avocado, Fresh

1 Teaspoon Vanilla, Pure

½ Teaspoon Pumpkin Pie Spice

Directions:

Combine all ingredients together until blended.

67. Cantaloupe Smoothie Bowl

Preparation Time: 5 Minutes

Cooking Time: 0 minutes

Serves: 2

Calories: 135

Protein: 3 Grams

Fat: 1 Gram

Carbs: 32 Grams

Ingredients:

¾ Cup carrot Juice

4 Cps Cantaloupe, Frozen & Cubed

Mellon Balls or Berries to Serve

Pinch Sea Salt

Directions:

Blend everything together until smooth.

68. Berry & Cauliflower Smoothie

Preparation Time: 10 Minutes

Cooking Time: 0 minutes

Serves: 2

Calories: 149

Protein: 3 Grams

Fat: 3 Grams

Carbs: 29 Grams

Ingredients:

1 Cup Riced Cauliflower, Frozen

1 Cup Banana, Sliced & Frozen

½ Cup Mixed Berries, Frozen

2 Cups Almond Milk, Unsweetened

2 Teaspoons Maple syrup, Pure & Optional

Directions:

Blend until mixed well.

69. Green Mango Smoothie

Preparation Time: 5 Minutes

Cooking Time: 0 minutes

Serves: 1

Calories: 417

Protein: 7.2 Grams

Fat: 2.8 Grams

Carbs: 102.8 Grams

Ingredients:

2 Cups Spinach

1-2 Cups Coconut Water

2 Mangos, Ripe, Peeled & Diced

Directions:

Blend everything together until smooth.

70. Chia Seed Smoothie

Preparation Time: 5 Minutes

Cooking Time: 0 minutes

Serves: 3

Calories: 477

Protein: 8 Grams

Fat: 29 Grams

Carbs: 57 Grams

Ingredients:

¼ Teaspoon Cinnamon

1 Tablespoon Ginger, Fresh & Grated

Pinch Cardamom

1 Tablespoon Chia Seeds

2 Medjool Dates, Pitted

1 Cup Alfalfa Sprouts

1 Cup Water

1 Banana

½ Cup Coconut Milk, Unsweetened

Directions:

Blend everything together until smooth.

71. Mango Smoothie

Preparation Time: 5 Minutes

Cooking Time: 0 minutes

Serves: 3

Calories: 376

Protein: 5 Grams

Fat: 2 Grams

Carbs: 95 Grams

Ingredients:

1 Carrot, Peeled & Chopped

1 Cup Strawberries

1 Cup Water

1 Cup Peaches, Chopped

1 Banana, Frozen & sliced

1 Cup Mango, Chopped

Directions:

Blend everything together until smooth.

Chapter 5 :Snacks and Desserts

72. Mango And Banana Shake

Preparation time: 10 mins

Cooking time: 0 mins

Servings: 2

Ingredients:

1 Banana, Sliced And Frozen

1 Cup Frozen Mango Chunks

1 Cup Almond Milk

1 Tbsp. Maple Syrup

1 Tsp Lime Juice

2-4 Raspberries For Topping

Mango Slice For Topping

Directions

In blender, pulse banana, mango with milk, maple syrup, lime juice until smooth but still thick Add more liquid if needed.

Pour shake into 2 bowls.Top with berries and mango slice.

Enjoy!

Nutrition: Protein: 5% 8 kcal Fat: 11% 18 kcal Carbohydrates: 85% 140 kcal

73. Avocado Toast With Flaxseeds

Preparation time: 5 mins.

Cooking time: 0 mins

Servings: 3

Ingredients:

3 slice of whole grain bread

1 large avocado, ripe

¼ cup chopped parsley

1 tbsp. flax seeds

1 tbsp. sesame seeds

1 tbsp. lime juice

Directions:

First, toast your piece of bread.

Remove the avocado seed.

Slice half avocado and mash half avocado with fork in bowl.

Spread mashed avocado on 2 toasted bread.

Place avocado slice on 1 toast.Top with flax seeds and sesame seeds.

Drizzle lime juice and chopped parsley on top.

Serve and enjoy!

Nutrition: Protein: 12% 31 kcal Fat: 49% 124 kcal Carbohydrates:

39% 98 kcal

74. Avocado Hummus

Preparation time: 10 mins

Cooking time:

Servings: 4

Ingredients

2 Ripe Avocados

½ Cup Coconut Cream

¼ Cup Sesame Paste

½ Lemon Juice

1 Tsp. Clove, Pressed

½ Tsp Ground Cumin

½ Tsp Salt

¼ Tsp Ground Black Pepper

Directions

Cut the avocado lengthways and remove seed from the fruit.

Put all ingredients in a blender or food processor and mix until

thoroughly smooth.Add more cream, lemon juice or water if you want to have a loosertexture.Adjust seasonings as needed.

Serve with naan and enjoy.

Nutrition: Protein: 6% 21 kcal Fat: 79% 289 kcal Carbohydrates:

16% 57 kcal

75. Plant Based Crispy Falafel

Preparation time: 20 mins

Cooking time: 30 mins

Servings: 8

Ingredients

1 tbsp. extra-virgin olive oil

1 cup dried chickpeas soaked for 24 hours in the refrigerator

1 cup cauliflower, chopped

½ cup red onion, chopped

½ cup packed fresh parsley

2 cloves garlic, quartered

1 tsp. sea salt

½ tsp. ground black pepper

½ tsp. ground cumin

¼ tsp. ground cinnamon

Directions

Preheat oven to 375° F.

In a food processor, mix chickpeas, cauliflower, onion, parsley, garlic,

salt, pepper, cumin seeds, cinnamon, and olive oil until mixture is

smooth.

Take 2 tbsps. of mixture and make the falafel into small patties.

Keep falafel on greased baking tray.

Bake falafel for about 25 to 30 minutes in preheated oven until

golden brown from both sides.

Once cooked remove from oven.

Serve hot fresh vegetable salad and enjoy!

Nutrition: Protein: 16% 19 kcal Fat: 24% 29 kcal Carbohydrates:

60% 71 kcal

76. Waffles With Almond Flour

Preparation time: 15 mins

Cooking time: 15 mins

Servings: 4

Ingredients

1 cup almond milk

2 tbsps. chia seeds

2 tsp lemon juice

4 tbsps. coconut oil

1/2 cup almond flour

2 tbsps. maple syrup

Cooking spray or cooking oil

Directions

Mix coconut milk with lemon juice in a mixing bowl.

Leave it for 5-8 minutes on room temperature to turn it into butter milk.

Once coconut milk is turned into butter milk, add chai seeds into milk and whisk together.

Add other ingredients in milk mixture and mix well.

Preheat a waffle iron and spray it with coconut oil spray.

Pour 2 tbsp. of waffle mixture into the waffle machine and cook until golden.

Top with some berries and serve hot.

Enjoy with black coffee!

Nutrition: Protein: 5% 15 kcal Fat: 71% 199 kcal Carbohydrates:

23% 66 kcal

77. Mint & Avocado Smoothie

Preparation time: 10 mins

Cooking time: 0 minutes

Servings: 2

Ingredients

1 cup coconut water

1/2 lemon juice

½ cup cucumber

1 cup mint. fresh

1/2 medium size avocado

I/2 tsp maple syrup

1 cup ice

Directions

Place all ingredients into a blender, cover lid and blend until smooth.

Blend on high speed until smoothie has fluffy texture.

Pour smoothie in glass and top with mint leaves.

Serve and enjoy!

Nutrition: Protein: 6% 7 kcal Fat: 51% 64 kcal Carbohydrates: 44%

55 kcal

78. Simple Banana Fritters

Preparation time: 15 mins

Cooking time: 20 mins

Servings: 8

Ingredients

4 Bananas

3 Tbsps. Maple Syrup

¼ Tsp. Cinnamon Powder

¼ Tsp. Nutmeg

1 Cup Coconut Flour

Directions

Preheat oven to 350° F.

Mash the bananas in a large mixing bowl along with maple syrup,

cinnamon, nutmeg powder and coconut flour.

Mix all the ingredients well.Take 2 tbsps. mixture and make small 1-inch-thick fritters from this mixture.Place fritters in greased baking tray.Bake fritters in preheated oven for about 10-15 minutes until golden from both sides. Once done, take them out of the oven.

Serve with coconut cream.

Enjoy!

Nutrition: Protein: 3% 3 kcal Fat: 28% 30 kcal Carbohydrates: 69%

75 kcal

79. Coconut And Blueberries Ice Cream

Preparation time: 5 mins

Cooking time: 0 mins

Servings: 4

Ingredients

1/4 Cup Coconut Cream

1 Tbsp. Maple Syrup

¼ Cup Coconut Flour

1 Cup Blueberries

¼ Cup Blueberries For Topping

Directions

Put ingredients into food processor and mix well on high speed.

Pour mixture in silicon molds and freeze in freezer for about 2-4 hours.

Once balls are set remove from freezer.

Top with berries.

Serve cold and enjoy!

Nutrition: Protein: 3% 4 kcal Fat: 40% 60 kcal Carbohydrates: 57% 86 kcal

80. Peach Crockpot Pudding

Preparation time: 15 mins

Cooking time: 4 hours

Servings: 6

Ingredients

2 Cups Sliced Peaches

1/4 Cup Maple Syrup

1/2 Tsp. Cinnamon Powder

2 Cups Coconut Milk

For Serving

½ Cup Coconut Cream

1 Oz. Coconut Flakes

Directions

Lightly grease the crockpot and place peaches in the bottom.

Add maple syrup, cinnamon powder and milk.Cover and cook on high for 4 hours.Once cooked remove from crockpot.

For serving pour coconut cream.Top with coconut flakes.

Serve and enjoy!

Nutrition: Protein: 3% 11 kcal Fat: 61% 230 kcal Carbohydrates: 36%

133 kcal

81. Raspberries & Cream Ice Cream

Preparation time: 5 mins

Cooking time: 0 mins

Servings: 4

Ingredients

2 Cups Raspberries

8 Oz. Coconut Cream

2 Tbsps. Coconut Flour

1 Tsp Maple Syrup

4-8 Raspberries For Filling

Directions

Mix all ingredients in food processor and blend until well combined.

Spoon mixture into silicone mold and with raspberries and freeze for about 4 hours.

Remove balls from freezer and pop them out of the molds.

Serve immediately and enjoy!

Nutrition: Protein: 5% 12 kcal Fat: 69% 170 kcal Carbohydrates: 26% 63 kcal

82. Healthy Chocolate Mousse

Preparation time: 5 mins

Cooking time: 0 mins

Servings: 2

Ingredients

1/2 Cup Coconut Milk

1 Tsp. Maple Syrup

1-3 Tbsps. Cocoa Powder

Pinch Instant Coffee

2 Tbsps. Coconut Cream

Blackberries For Topping

Directions

Heat up coconut milk and maple syrup until it just begins to simmer.

Add cocoa and coffee in milk mixture.Add cream to same mixture and whip until relatively stiff peaks form.

Transfer to a serving glass.

Chill the mousse in freezer for 2-3 hours.

Top with some berries and spoon of coconut cream.

Enjoy!

Nutrition: Protein: 3% 7 kcal Fat: 83% 163 kcal Carbohydrates: 13%

26 kcal

83. Coconut Rice With Mangos

Preparation time: 15 mins

Cooking time: 40 mins

Servings: 6

Ingredients

2 Cups Coconut Milk

1-1/2 Cups Coconut Flakes

1/4 Cup Maple Syrup

1 Mango Sliced

Directions

Heat saucepan over high heat.

Add coconut milk and bring it to boil.

Stir in coconut flakes and maple syrup.

Cover and cook on low heat for about 15 minutes or until liquid is completely dried.

Pour coconut rice in plate.

Serve with mango slice and enjoy.

Nutrition: Protein: 3% 8 kcal Fat: 69% 185 kcal Carbohydrates: 28% 75 kcal

84. Nori Snack Rolls

Preparation Time: 5 minutes

Cooking time: 10 minutes

Servings: 4 rolls

Ingredients

2 tablespoons almond, cashew, peanut, or others nut butter

2 tablespoons tamari, or soy sauce

4 standard nori sheets

1 mushroom, sliced

1 tablespoon pickled ginger

½ cup grated carrots

Directions

Preparing the Ingredients.

Preheat the oven to 350°F.

Mix together the nut butter and tamari until smooth and very thick.

Lay out a nori sheet, rough side up, the long way.

Spread a thin line of the tamari mixture on the far end of the nori sheet, from side to side. Lay the mushroom slices, ginger, and carrots in a line at the other end (the end closest to you).

Fold the vegetables inside the nori, rolling toward the tahini mixture, which will seal the roll. Repeat to make 4 rolls.

Put on a baking sheet and bake for 8 to 10 minutes, or until the rolls are slightly browned and crispy at the ends. Let the rolls cool for a few minutes, then slice each roll into 3 smaller pieces.

Nutrition: Calories: 79; Total fat: 5g; Carbs: 6g; Fiber: 2g; Protein: 4g

85. Risotto Bites

Preparation Time: 15 minutes

Cooking time: 20 minutes

Servings: 12 bites

Ingredients

½ cup panko bread crumbs

1 teaspoon paprika

1 teaspoon chipotle powder or ground cayenne pepper

1½ cups cold Green Pea Risotto

Nonstick cooking spray

Directions

Preparing the Ingredients.

Preheat the oven to 425°F.

Line a baking sheet with parchment paper.

On a large plate, combine the panko, paprika, and chipotle powder.
Set aside.

Roll 2 tablespoons of the risotto into a ball.

Gently roll in the bread crumbs, and place on the prepared baking
sheet. Repeat to make a total of 12 balls.

Spritz the tops of the risotto bites with nonstick cooking spray and
bake for 15 to 20 minutes, until they begin to brown. Cool completely

before storing in a large airtight container in a single layer (add a piece of parchment paper for a second layer) or in a plastic freezer bag.

Nutrition: Calories: 100; Fat: 2g; Protein: 6g; Carbohydrates: 17g; Fiber: 5g; Sugar: 2g; Sodium: 165 mg

86. Jicama and Guacamole

Preparation Time: 15 minutes

Cooking time: 0 minutes

Servings: 4

Ingredients

juice of 1 lime, or 1 tablespoon prepared lime juice

2 hass avocados, peeled, pits removed, and cut into cubes

½ teaspoon sea salt

½ red onion, minced

1 garlic clove, minced

¼ cup chopped cilantro (optional)

1 jicama bulb, peeled and cut into matchsticks

Directions

Preparing the Ingredients.

In a medium bowl, squeeze the lime juice over the top of the avocado and sprinkle with salt.

Lightly mash the avocado with a fork. Stir in the onion, garlic, and cilantro, if using.

Serve with slices of jicama to dip in guacamole.

To store, place plastic wrap over the bowl of guacamole and refrigerate. The guacamole will keep for about 2 days.

87. Curried Tofu "Egg Salad" Pitas

Preparation Time: 15 minutes

Cooking time: 0 minutes

Servings: 4 sandwiches

Ingredients

1 pound extra-firm tofu, drained and patted dry

$1/$ cup vegan mayonnaise, homemade or store-bought

$1/$ cup chopped mango chutney, homemade or store-bought

2 teaspoons Dijon mustard

1 tablespoon hot or mild curry powder

1 teaspoon salt

$1/$ teaspoon ground cayenne

¾ cup shredded carrots

2 celery ribs, minced

$1/$ cup minced red onion

8 small Boston or other soft lettuce leaves

4 (7-inch) whole wheat pita breads, halved

Directions

Crumble the tofu and place it in a large bowl. Add the mayonnaise, chutney, mustard, curry powder, salt, and cayenne, and stir well until thoroughly mixed.

Add the carrots, celery, and onion and stir to combine. Refrigerate for 30 minutes to allow the flavors to blend.

Tuck a lettuce leaf inside each pita pocket, spoon some tofu mixture on top of the lettuce, and serve.

88. Garden Salad Wraps

Preparation Time: 15 minutes

Cooking time: 10 minutes

Servings: 4 wraps

Ingredients

6 tablespoons olive oil

1 pound extra-firm tofu, drained, patted dry, and cut into ½ -inch

strips

1 tablespoon soy sauce

½ cup apple cider vinegar

1 teaspoon yellow or spicy brown mustard

½ teaspoon salt

½ teaspoon freshly ground black pepper

3 cups shredded romaine lettuce

3 ripe Roma tomatoes, finely chopped

1 large carrot, shredded

1 medium English cucumber, peeled and chopped

½ cup minced red onion

½ cup sliced pitted green olives

4 (10-inch) whole-grain flour tortillas or lavash flatbread

Directions

In a large skillet, heat 2 tablespoons of the oil over medium heat.
Add the tofu and cook until golden brown, about 10 minutes. Sprinkle
with soy sauce and set aside to cool.

In a small bowl, combine the vinegar, mustard, salt, and pepper with
the remaining 4 tablespoons oil, stirring to blend well. Set aside.

In a large bowl, combine the lettuce, tomatoes, carrot, cucumber,
onion, and olives. Pour on the dressing and toss to coat.

To assemble wraps, place 1 tortilla on a work surface and spread
with about one-quarter of the salad. Place a few strips of tofu on the
tortilla and roll up tightly. Slice in half 76.

89. Tamari Toasted Almonds

Preparation Time: 2 minutes

Cooking time: 8 minutes

Servings: ½ cup

Ingredients

½ cup raw almonds, or sunflower seeds

2 tablespoons tamari, or soy sauce

1 teaspoon toasted sesame oil

Directions

Preparing the Ingredients.

Heat a dry skillet to medium-high heat, then add the almonds, stirring very frequently to keep them from burning. Once the almonds are toasted, 7 to 8 minutes for almonds, or 3 to 4 minutes for sunflower seeds, pour the tamari and sesame oil into the hot skillet and stir to coat.

You can turn off the heat, and as the almonds cool the tamari mixture will stick to and dry on the nuts.

Per Serving (1 tablespoon) Calories: 89; Total fat: 8g; Carbs: 3g; Fiber: 2g; Protein: 4g

90. Avocado And Tempeh Bacon Wraps

Preparation Time: 10 minutes

Cooking time: 8 minutes

Servings: 4 wraps

Ingredients

2 tablespoons olive oil

8 ounces tempeh bacon, homemade or store-bought

4 (10-inch) soft flour tortillas or lavash flatbread

⅟ cup vegan mayonnaise, homemade or store-bought

4 large lettuce leaves

2 ripe Hass avocados, pitted, peeled, and cut into ⅟ -inch slices

1 large ripe tomato, cut into ⅟ -inch slices

Directions

In a large skillet, heat the oil over medium heat. Add the tempeh

bacon and cook until browned on both sides, about 8 minutes.

Remove from the heat and set aside.

Place 1 tortilla on a work surface. Spread with some of the

mayonnaise and one-fourth of the lettuce and tomatoes.

Pit, peel, and thinly slice the avocado and place the slices on top of

the tomato. Add the reserved tempeh bacon and roll up tightly.

Repeat with remaining Ingredients and serve.

91. Kale Chips

Preparation Time: 5 minutes

Cooking time: 25 minutes

Servings: 2

Ingredients

1 large bunch kale

1 tablespoon extra-virgin olive oil

½ teaspoon chipotle powder

½ teaspoon smoked paprika

¼ teaspoon salt

Directions

Preparing the Ingredients.

Preheat the oven to 275°F.

Line a large baking sheet with parchment paper. In a large bowl, stem the kale and tear it into bite-size pieces. Add the olive oil, chipotle powder, smoked paprika, and salt.

Toss the kale with tongs or your hands, coating each piece well.

Spread the kale over the parchment paper in a single layer.

Bake for 25 minutes, turning halfway through, until crisp.

Cool for 10 to 15 minutes before dividing and storing in 2 airtight containers.

Nutrition: Calories: 144; Fat: 7g; Protein: 5g; Carbohydrates: 18g;

Fiber: 3g; Sugar: 0g; Sodium: 363mg.

CPSIA information can be obtained
at www.ICGtesting.com
Printed in the USA
LVHW031144281220
675195LV00005B/51